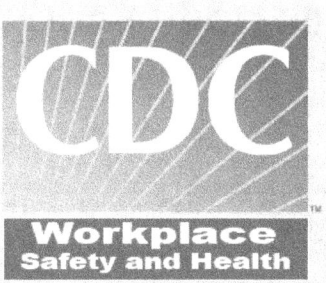

Comparison of Mold Exposures, Work-related Symptoms, and Visual Contrast Sensitivity between Employees at a Severely Water-damaged School and Employees at a School without Significant Water Damage

Gregory Thomas, MD, MS
Nancy Clark Burton, PhD, MPH, CIH
Charles Mueller, MS
Elena Page, MD, MPH

Health Hazard Evaluation Report
HETA 2005-0135-3116
Alcee Fortier Senior High School
New Orleans, Louisiana
September 2010

DEPARTMENT OF HEALTH AND HUMAN SERVICES
Centers for Disease Control and Prevention

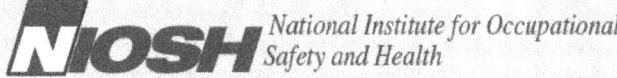
National Institute for Occupational
Safety and Health

The employer shall post a copy of this report for a period of 30 calendar days at or near the workplace(s) of affected employees. The employer shall take steps to insure that the posted determinations are not altered, defaced, or covered by other material during such period. [37 FR 23640, November 7, 1972, as amended at 45 FR 2653, January 14, 1980].

CONTENTS

ABBREVIATIONS

μg/dL	Micrograms per deciliter
μg/g	Micrograms per gram
μm	Micrometer
ACGIH®	American Conference of Governmental Industrial Hygienists
AFSHS	Alcee Fortier Senior High School
AIHA	American Industrial Hygiene Association
ANSI	American National Standards Institute
ASHRAE	American Society of Heating, Refrigerating, and Air-Conditioning Engineers
BLL	Blood lead level
CDC	Centers for Disease Control and Prevention
CO_2	Carbon dioxide
CFR	Code of Federal Regulations
CFU/m^3	Colony forming units per cubic meter
cpd	Cycles per degree
ERMI	Environmental relative moldiness index
F A.C.T.®	Functional acuity contrast test
HHE	Health hazard evaluation
HEPA	High-efficiency particulate air
HUD	U.S. Department of Housing and Urban Development
HVAC	Heating, ventilating, and air-conditioning
IEQ	Indoor environmental quality
IOM	Institute of Medicine
LASIK	Laser-assisted in situ keratomileusis
Lpm	Liters per minute
Ls^{-1}	Liters per second
MEA	Malt extract agar
MSQPCR	Mold specific quantitative polymerase chain reaction
NAICS	North American Industry Classification System
NIOSH	National Institute for Occupational Safety and Health
NOPS	New Orleans Public School
OEL	Occupational exposure limit
OSHA	Occupational Safety and Health Administration
PEL	Permissible exposure limit
ppm	Parts per million
RH	Relative humidity
U.S. EPA	United States Environmental Protection Agency
VCS	Visual contrast sensitivity
VOC	Volatile organic compound
WHO	World Health Organization
WHHS	Walnut Hills High School

The National Institute for Occupational Safety and Health (NIOSH) received a request for a health hazard evaluation at the Alcee Fortier Senior High School (AFSHS) in New Orleans, Louisiana. Employees were concerned about exposures to mold and lead paint. The employees reported difficulty breathing, chronic sinusitis, and immune system problems.

What NIOSH Did

- We evaluated the school in April 2005 and again in May 2005.

- We also evaluated Walnut Hills High School (WHHS) in Cincinnati, Ohio, in February 2006. This school is about the same age as AFSHS, but has no history of water damage or mold contamination. We compared the two schools.

- We looked for signs of water damage and mold in both schools. We also reviewed industrial hygiene reports for both schools.

- We collected air, bulk, and surface samples for mold in the AFSHS and WHHS buildings. We collected bulk paint samples for lead at AFSHS but not at WHHS because there was no peeling paint.

- We looked at the ventilation systems and checked the moisture levels in the walls at both schools. We also measured carbon dioxide, temperature, and relative humidity levels in both schools.

- We surveyed employees at both schools. We asked about their work, medical history, and work-related health concerns.

- We conducted visual contrast sensitivity tests on employees at both schools.

What NIOSH Found

- We found mold and moisture problems throughout AFSHS. Only one area at WHHS was identified with an ongoing moisture problem.

- We found lead in the bulk paint samples from AFSHS.

- The carbon dioxide, temperature, and relative humidity levels were acceptable at AFSHS. Carbon dioxide measurements were elevated in some classrooms at WHHS.

- Employees at AFSHS had significantly higher prevalences of symptoms than employees at WHHS. These included rashes and nasal, lower respiratory, constitutional, and neurobehavioral symptoms.

- We found significantly lower visual contrast sensitivity test results for AFSHS compared with WHHS employees, indicating that mild visual changes had occurred.

What New Orleans Public School District Administrators Can Do

Because AFSHS is now a private school and has been renovated, general recommendations for maintaining good indoor environmental quality are provided to the New Orleans Public School District for use at all schools.

- Follow a routine maintenance schedule for all ventilation systems.

- Implement an indoor environmental quality management plan.

- Address existing moisture problems, and have an action plan to address future occurrences.

- Set up a health and safety committee with school administration and employees. Ensure the group has adequate time and money to function effectively.

What WHHS Administrators Can Do

- Make sure adequate amounts of outdoor air are supplied to classrooms.

- Address moisture problems in the band rooms and remediate existing mold contamination.

What Employees Can Do

- Report work-related health concerns to school officials.

- See an experienced occupational medicine physician if you have health concerns that may be related to your work.

- Become active in the safety and health committee.

Summary

NIOSH investigators compared work-related symptoms and VCS between employees at a school with severe water damage and those at a school without significant water damage. Employees at the water-damaged school had higher prevalences of work-related rashes and nasal, lower respiratory, and constitutional symptoms than those at the school without significant water damage. VCS values across all spatial frequencies were lower among employees at the water-damaged school. Further studies are needed to determine what factors could be responsible for the VCS findings and whether they have any clinical significance for affected individuals. The building problems at AFSHS need to be addressed; recommendations to prevent water damage and microbial growth and for remediation in NOPS and WHHS are provided in this report.

On January 18, 2005, NIOSH received a request for an HHE at AFSHS in New Orleans, Louisiana. Employees submitted the request because of concerns about exposure to mold and lead paint in their school building. Employees reported a variety of health effects, including difficulty breathing, chronic sinusitis, immune system problems, nosebleeds, skin rashes, irregular menses, headaches, irritable bowel syndrome, and nausea.

We visited AFSHS on April 18–19, 2005. During informal interviews, employees reported possible work-related symptoms, some of which were consistent with symptoms reported by people working in water-damaged buildings. The building had obvious microbial contamination, so we decided that further evaluation was needed. On May 23–24, 2005, we returned to New Orleans for a follow-up evaluation. During this visit we administered a work history and health symptom questionnaire. We also conducted VCS testing using the F A.C.T.® handheld chart. VCS testing measures the subjects' ability to determine changes in alternating light and dark bands of varying intensity. Performance on this test has been adversely associated with exposure to neurotoxins such as solvents and lead among many other conditions and exposures such as aging, certain eye conditions, alcohol and medication use, and depression. We used VCS testing for this evaluation to determine if it could serve as a biomarker of effect for occupants who experience adverse effects from a water-damaged building. We also collected environmental samples for culturable and aerosolized fungal spores and measured IEQ parameters (CO_2, temperature, and RH). We performed a similar evaluation at WHHS in Cincinnati, Ohio, on February 27–29, 2006. WHHS had no history of ongoing water intrusion or mold growth.

Of 119 employees at AFSHS, 95 (80%) participated in the evaluation. Of 165 employees at WHHS, 110 (67%) participated. Participants at both schools were similar in sex, age, history of psychiatric disease, atopy (the predisposition to allergic disease), smoking history, and having mold or moisture problems in their homes.

Employees at AFSHS had higher prevalences of work-related cough, wheezing, or whistling in the chest; chest tightness; unusual shortness of breath; sinus problems; sore or dry throat; frequent sneezing; stuffy nose; runny nose; fever or sweats; aching all over; unusual tiredness or fatigue; headache; difficulty concentrating; confusion or disorientation; trouble remembering things; change in sleep patterns; and rash, dermatitis, or eczema on the face, neck, or arms than employees at WHHS. At each school, 13 employees reported currently having asthma. A significantly higher percent of the asthmatics at AFSHS reported their asthma was worse at work.

Monocular and binocular VCS values were significantly lower at all spatial frequencies among AFSHS employees. A significantly higher percentage of employees at AFSHS had scores that fell below the average performance for 90% of the population compared to the results found among employees at WHHS.

Actively growing *Cladosporium* was found on the walls of AFSHS. Mold was found in all three MSQPCR air samples with *C. sphaerospermum* being the most prevalent. The vacuum dust samples detected 32 of the 35 fungal species tested. The culturable air samples showed that *Cladosporium* and *Pencillium* were the most prevalent genera both inside and outside the school. *Aspergillus* species were detected in inside samples but not in outside air samples. The spore trap samples showed that *Cladosporium* was the prevalent genera both inside and outside the school with the exception of Room 316.

No fungal growth was detected on six of eight sticky tape samples collected at WHHS. One had a trace of hyphae, and the other showed a few *Aspergillus/Pencillium*-like spores and a trace of hyphae. Both were from the band room. Air samples analyzed with MSQPCR showed low counts for inside samples compared to outside samples. The culturable and spore trap air samples collected inside and outside WHHS were comparable in terms of both counts and genera ranking. CO_2 concentrations were elevated in some classrooms.

We determined that a health hazard existed at AFSHS. Employees had significantly higher prevalences of rashes and nasal, lower respiratory, and constitutional symptoms than employees at WHHS. The prevalences of several neurobehavioral symptoms were also significantly higher. VCS values across all spatial frequencies were lower in the employees at AFSHS. Further studies are needed to determine what factors could be responsible for the VCS findings and whether they have any clinical significance for affected individuals. The building problems at AFSHS need to be addressed; recommendations to prevent water damage and microbial growth and for remediation in NOPS and WHHS are provided in this report.

Keywords: NAICS 611110 (Elementary and Secondary Schools), indoor environmental quality, IEQ, ERMI, mold, lead, F.A.C.T., visual contrast sensitivity

On January 18, 2005, NIOSH received an employee request for an HHE at the AFSHS in New Orleans, Louisiana, because of concerns about exposure to mold and lead paint in their school building. Employees reported a variety of health effects, including difficulty breathing, chronic sinusitis, immune system problems, nosebleeds, skin rashes, irregular menses, headaches, irritable bowel syndrome, and nausea.

After review of the request and telephone consultations with the requestor and administrative representatives of AFSHS, an initial site visit was made on April 18–19, 2005. An opening conference was held at the AFSHS library with school administrators, school medical personnel, and local representatives of the NOPS teachers' union. Following the opening conference, a walk-through of the school was conducted and confidential, open-ended interviews were held with AFSHS employees. In addition, preliminary environmental sampling (collection of tape samples for microscopic analysis for fungal spores, collection of bulk paint samples for lead analysis, and use of a moisture meter to qualitatively assess wall moisture levels) was performed in the school building. Among the symptoms employees reported were possible work-related respiratory symptoms consistent with symptoms reported in other water-damaged buildings. They also reported neurobehavioral symptoms such as difficulty concentrating, irritability, and trouble remembering things.

On May 23–24, 2005, we returned to New Orleans for a follow-up evaluation at AFSHS to administer a work and health history questionnaire and to conduct VCS testing. We used VCS testing for this evaluation to determine if it could serve as a biomarker of effect for occupants who experience adverse effects from a water-damaged building. A biomarker is an indicator that signals an event or condition in a biological system or sample and gives a measure of exposure, effect, or susceptibility. A biomarker of effect is associated with an established or possible health impairment or disease. We also collected environmental samples for culturable and aerosolized fungal spores and measured IEQ parameters (CO_2, temperature, and RH).

VCS testing has been reported as useful in "diagnosing" and monitoring treatment of "biotoxin-related illness" among individuals exposed to water-damaged buildings [Shoemaker and House 2005; Shoemaker and House 2006]. "Biotoxin-related illness" is not a generally accepted medical condition, and reportedly consists of multiorgan system symptoms, among which neurobehavioral symptoms are prominent. Interpretation of these studies is hampered by methodological limitations, including a nonrepresentative sample, medical conditions that often present with multiple system symptoms (fibromyalgia and chronic fatigue syndrome), the lack of a comparison group, and poor exposure characterization. These limitations could account for the lower VCS values in the participants of these studies, rather than illness from exposure to water-damaged buildings.

VCS has been documented to be adversely affected by exposure to toxic substances that affect the central nervous system such as solvents [Frenette et al. 1991; Broadwell et al. 1995; Schreiber et al. 2002; Boeckelmann and Pfister 2003; Gong et al. 2003; Hitchcock et al. 2003]. Some of these studies have noted deficits in the midspatial frequencies [Broadwell et al. 1995; Schreiber et al. 2002] while others have documented deficits across all frequencies [Frenette et al. 1991; Gong et al. 2003]. A number of visual conditions also affect VCS, including cataracts, glaucoma, LASIK, retinopathy, and dry eye. Recently, patients with major depression have been found to have worse contrast discrimination than controls [Bubl et al. 2009]. VCS is adversely affected by aging, alcohol use, and attention deficit hyperactivity disorder [Pearson and Timney 1999; Nomura et al. 2003; Bartgis et al. 2009].

We planned a third visit to New Orleans to perform similar testing at a local school that did not have water intrusion or mold growth. However, damage from Hurricane Katrina and the subsequent flooding prevented access to an appropriate comparison school in New Orleans.

We requested and were granted access to WHHS in Cincinnati, Ohio, for comparison. This large public school is similar in age to AFSHS. The school did not have a history of extensive or ongoing water intrusion or mold growth. We made a site visit to WHHS from February 27–29, 2006. An environmental evaluation was performed, a questionnaire was administered, and VCS testing was conducted on all participants at WHHS.

Facility Descriptions

Alcee Fortier Senior High School

At the time of the 2005 site visits, AFSHS was one of 130 schools in the NOPS district. It was an inner city high school on the western edge of New Orleans. The school had 119 staff members and 850 students in the 9th through 12th grades. A school nurse was on site, and custodial and ventilation maintenance services were contracted out.

The AFSHS building was constructed in 1929 and opened in 1930. The building was a large masonry (stone and marble) four-story structure with a flat membrane/gravel roof. The building was originally designed with a natural ventilation system using large exterior windows and windows at the top of the interior walls adjacent to the hallways to provide cross-ventilation. In 2002, individual ventilation units (Scholar QV™, Marvair Cordele, Georgia) were installed in each classroom and hallway. Each unit was placed on an exterior wall; the ventilation unit's louvered outside air intake replaced an existing window. The ventilation systems were powered off during evenings and weekends to save energy. Ceiling fans were used in the classrooms to circulate air. The classrooms had hardwood floors, and the hallways had tile floors. The band room had a separate HVAC system.

Walnut Hills High School

WHHS was built in 1930. The main building was a stone and brick structure with primarily concrete floors. It had no significant history of water incursion or mold problems, and was chosen as a comparison to AFSHS based on ease of access and age of the building. The ventilation system consisted of steam heat in the winter and air conditioning for cooling. A roof leak and mold contamination in the library were remediated in 1995. Evidence of a past roof leak was seen in and around the band/music room located under the school patio. The art and science building, added in 1999, showed no evidence of moisture incursion. This building had an independent, ducted HVAC system.

Review of Previous IEQ Evaluations of the AFSHS Building

Review of reports furnished by AFSHS included citations dated from 1997 to 2002 by the State Office of Public Health, reports from the State of Louisiana Department of Health and Hospitals, and the Orleans Parish School Board Request for Repairs and Alterations. These documents primarily allude to problems with extensive peeling paint (some of which was lead-based) on walls and ceilings, noninsulated pipes, mold remediation projects, and broken windows.

Medical

All employees at both schools were invited to participate in the evaluation. Each participant gave full informed consent and filled out a questionnaire about his or her age, medical history, work history, exposure to mold or moisture in the home, and symptoms experienced during the last month while working in the school. These included upper respiratory and mucus membrane, lower respiratory, constitutional, neurobehavioral, and dermal symptoms. If the participant reported having the symptom during the previous month while in the school and that it improved or went away on days off work, the symptom was considered work-related. VCS testing was conducted using the F A.C.T. handheld chart [Ginsburg 1993]. We also measured visual acuity with a handheld Snellen chart. Results from persons with visual acuity of 20/50 or less were removed from further analysis. The tests were conducted monocularly and binocularly under standard daylight illumination in the library of each school. A light meter was used to ensure that ambient illumination met the requirements specified for the F A.C.T. handheld chart (between 68 and 239 candelas per square meter). Participants who used corrective lenses were asked to wear them during testing. Additional information concerning VCS and the statistical methods used for this report is located in Appendix A.

Environmental

During the first site visit at AFSHS on April 18–19, 2005, sticky tape samples from surfaces were collected throughout the school for microscopic fungal analysis. Vacuum dust samples were analyzed for the presence of fungal species using a DNA-based method called MSQPCR [Haugland et al. 2002]. A nondestructive moisture meter was used to qualitatively assess the interior wall moisture levels. To address requestors' concerns over the potential for lead exposures from peeling paint, paint samples were collected and analyzed for lead.

During the second site visit to AFSHS, a more detailed environmental evaluation was conducted. Air samples for culturable fungi were collected using Andersen N-6 samplers (Thermo Electron Corporation, Waltham, Massachusetts) with MEA agar plates. Spore trap samples were collected using Air-o-Cell® samplers (Zefon International, Inc., Ocala, Florida). Measurements of CO_2, temperature, and RH, as indicators of comfort, were taken throughout the workday. Additional sticky tape samples were collected for microscopic fungal analysis, and one additional paint sample was collected and analyzed for lead. A more detailed description of the sampling methods can be found in Appendix A. Information on OELs and health effects for IEQ, mold, and lead is provided in Appendix B.

A similar environmental protocol for mold testing was used for the WHHS evaluation. Environmental samples collected included sticky tape samples for microscopic fungal analysis and air samples for culturable fungi, MSQPCR, and spore trap analyses. Measurements of CO_2, temperature, and RH were made throughout the workday. Additional information concerning the sampling protocol is given in Appendix A.

RESULTS

Of 119 AFSHS employees, 95 (80%) participated in the evaluation; 65 were teachers or teaching aides. The rest were administrative personnel, food service staff, janitorial staff, security staff, nurses, counselors, and speech therapists. Of 165 WHHS employees, 110 (67%) participated; 73 were teachers, 21 were administrative personnel, and the rest were food service staff, janitorial staff, security staff, nurses, counselors, and speech therapists. Participants at both schools were similar in sex, age, history of psychiatric disorder, atopy (the predisposition to allergic disease), smoking history, and having mold or moisture problems in their home. A significantly higher percentage of AFSHS employees had hypertension, which may adversely affect VCS. A significantly higher percentage of WHHS employees reported head injuries. The median number of alcoholic drinks among WHHS employees was higher than those at AFSHS. Alcohol intake and head injuries may also adversely affect VCS. The prevalence of current asthma was very similar between schools. Demographic information is presented in Table 1.

Table 1. Selected characteristics of participants, by school

Variable	AFSHS n=91–95*	WHHS n=98–109*
Age (mean)	46 years	48 years
Tenure (median)	4 years	8 years
Number of alcoholic beverages in the past 30 days (median)	0	3
	number (%)	number (%)
Female	49 (52)	59 (55)
Mold or moisture problem at home	6 (6)	9 (8)
Ever had asthma	20 (21)	13 (12)
Physician diagnosed asthma	19 (20)	12 (11)
Currently have asthma	13 (14)	13 (12)
Atopy[†]	69 (73)	75 (69)
Diabetes	8 (8)	4 (4)
Hypertension	37 (39)	28 (26)
Physician-diagnosed anxiety	15 (16)	15 (14)
Physician-diagnosed depression	15 (16)	17 (16)
Physician-diagnosed obsessive compulsive disorder	1 (1)	2 (2)
Physician-diagnosed bipolar disorder	3 (3)	1 (1)
History of eye surgery	3 (3)	10 (9)
History of head injury	10 (11)	23 (21)
Ever smoked cigars, cigarettes, or pipes	32 (34)	35 (33)

*Denominators vary due to missing information
[†]Atopy is a self-reported history of asthma, allergic rhinitis or hay fever, or eczema. Atopy signifies a predisposition to allergic disease.

Employees at AFSHS had higher prevalences of work-related rash and lower respiratory, upper respiratory, constitutional, and neurobehavioral symptoms compared to WHHS employees (Table 2). All but dry or irritated eyes, nosebleeds, irritability, and depression were statistically significantly higher. Thirteen employees at each school reported currently having asthma, but 69% of the asthmatics at AFSHS reported their asthma was worse at work, compared to 23% at WHHS (*P*=0.02). We removed employees with current asthma from our analyses for lower respiratory symptoms and found that AFSHS employees still had significantly higher prevalences of work-related cough (*P*<0.01), wheezing or whistling in the chest, (*P*<0.01), chest tightness (*P*<0.01), and unusual shortness of breath (*P*<0.01). In previous studies we have used the presence of work-related wheezing or whistling in the chest, or two of the following three symptoms: cough, chest tightness, or unusual shortness of breath to define symptoms consistent with work-related asthma. Excluding those who reported current, physician-diagnosed asthma, 20 employees at AFSHS met the definition of symptoms consistent with work-related asthma and, therefore, may have undiagnosed or unrecognized asthma.

Table 2. Prevalence of work-related symptoms in the last month, by school

Symptom	AFSHS n= 81–88*	WHHS n=102–107*	Prevalence Ratio (95% Confidence Interval)	P value
	number (%)	number (%)		
Lower Respiratory				
Cough	35 (43)	11 (10)	4.16 (2.26, 7.68)	<0.01
Wheezing or whistling in chest	19 (23)	2 (2)	12.13 (2.91, 50.62)	<0.01
Chest tightness	22 (27)	0	+inf (7.69, +inf)†	<0.01
Unusual shortness of breath	19 (24)	4 (4)	6.22 (2.20, 17.56)	<0.01
Upper Respiratory				
Sinus problems	27 (33)	14 (13)	2.44 (1.37, 4.35)	<0.01
Dry or irritated eyes	16 (20)	12 (11)	1.72 (0.86, 3.44)	0.12
Nosebleeds	3 (4)	1 (1)	3.70 (0.53, 47.02)	0.33
Sore or dry throat	21 (24)	13 (13)	1.95 (1.04, 3.67)	0.03
Frequent sneezing	17 (20)	4 (4)	5.23 (1.83, 14.96)	<0.01
Stuffy nose	25 (29)	10 (10)	3.09 (1.57, 6.07)	<0.01
Runny nose	22 (25)	7 (7)	3.87 (1.73, 8.62)	<0.01
Constitutional				
Fever or sweats	14 (16)	4 (4)	4.10 (1.40, 12.01)	<0.01
Aching all over	12 (14)	4 (4)	3.71 (1.24, 11.08)	0.01
Unusual tiredness or fatigue	25 (31)	18 (17)	1.78 (1.04, 3.03)	0.03
Headache	30 (35)	21 (20)	1.74 (1.08, 2.81)	0.02
Neurobehavioral				
Difficulty concentrating	15 (18)	4 (4)	4.63 (1.60, 13.44)	<0.01
Confusion or disorientation	8 (10)	2 (2)	5.05 (1.25, 29.56)	0.02
Trouble remembering things	15 (17)	5 (5)	3.59 (1.36, 9.47)	<0.01
Irritability	19 (22)	15 (14)	1.51 (0.82, 2.80)	0.18
Depression	6 (7)	2 (2)	3.74 (0.87, 20.82)	0.14
Change in sleep patterns	16 (19)	4 (4)	4.99 (1.73, 14.37)	<0.01
Rash, dermatitis, or eczema (on face, neck, arms, or hands)	12 (14)	4 (4)	3.70 (1.24, 11.06)	0.01

*Denominators vary because of missing information.
†Positive infinity or undefined

Fifteen individuals were excluded from analyses of VCS because of conditions that could affect their VCS such as glaucoma, cataract, LASIK surgery, or retinal surgery (4 from AFSHS and 11 from WHHS). Eighteen left eyes (8 from AFSHS and 10 from WHHS) and 19 right eyes (8 from AFSHS and 11 from WHHS) were excluded because near visual acuity was $\geq 20/50$. Three individuals were excluded from analyses because their binocular near visual acuity was $\geq 20/50$ (two from AFSHS and one from WHHS). Near monocular and binocular visual acuity did not differ significantly between the remaining WHHS and AFSHS employees who were included in the analyses. Monocular and binocular VCS values were significantly lower at all spatial frequencies among AFSHS employees ($P<0.01$). We repeated the analyses excluding diabetics, and results were similar. We compared VCS values between schools among only hypertensives, and again among only nonhypertensives. We found lower values at all frequencies among AFSHS employees in both groups, although the differences were not statistically significant among the hypertensives at spatial frequencies 1.5 cpd ($P=0.12$) or 18

Table 3. Prevalence of visual contrast sensitivity scores below 90% of the population

	AFSHS n=80 number (%)	WHHS n=81 number (%)	P value
Left Eye (cpd)			
1.5	10 (13)	1 (1)	<0.01
3	11 (14)	1 (1)	<0.01
6	23 (29)	4 (5)	<0.01
12	23 (29)	3 (4)	<0.01
18	22 (28)	2 (3)	<0.01
Right Eye (cpd)			
1.5	7 (9)	0 (0)	<0.01
3	10 (13)	1 (1)	<0.01
6	21 (26)	2 (3)	<0.01
12	22 (28)	4 (5)	<0.01
18	23 (29)	6 (7)	<0.01
Both Eyes (cpd)	n=86	n=95	
1.5	0 (0)	0 (0)	NA
3	2 (2)	0 (0)	0.22
6	11 (13)	1 (1)	<0.01
12	10 (12)	2 (2)	0.01
18	11 (13)	1 (1)	<0.01

cpd (*P*=0.07) in the left eye or spatial frequencies 12 cpd (*P*=0.12) and 18 cpd (*P*=0.16) binocularly among nonhypertensives. A significantly higher percentage of employees at AFSHS had scores at all spatial frequencies in the both the right eye and left eye that fell below the average performance for 90% of the population (i.e., in the lower 10th percentile) than employees at WHHS (Table 3).

Because some people with allergies and asthma report a variety of neurobehavioral symptoms, including fatigue, sleepiness, poor concentration, poor work or school performance, and irritability, and studies have found objective evidence of cognitive impairment in these persons, we assessed whether VCS decrements were associated with upper or lower respiratory symptoms (Table 4). We combined work-related symptoms into the following symptom complexes: upper respiratory (sinus problems, dry or irritated eyes, nosebleeds, sore or dry throat, frequent sneezing, stuffy nose, or runny nose) and lower respiratory (cough, wheezing or whistling in the chest, chest tightness, or unusual shortness of breath). Persons reporting one or more symptom in a given symptom complex were considered to have that work-related symptom complex. Persons reporting one or more lower respiratory symptom had significantly lower mean VCS values at all spatial frequencies than those reporting no lower respiratory symptoms.

Table 4. Comparison of binocular VCS values between those with and without the symptom complex

Work-related Symptom Complex	Spatial Frequency (cycles per degree)	Both Schools* (*P* value) n=159–164
	1.5	<0.01
	3	<0.01
Upper Respiratory	6	0.07
	12	0.15
	18	0.09
	1.5	<0.01
	3	<0.01
Lower Respiratory	6	<0.01
	12	<0.01
	18	<0.01

*Indicates all findings in anticipated direction (i.e., mean VCS scores were lower for those with symptom complex)

Environmental

Alcee Fortier Senior High School

Of the sixteen sticky tape samples, 15 showed the presence of actively growing *Cladosporium* in numerous to massive amounts of growth on the walls of the school at the time of the site visits (Table C1). *Cladosporium*, a known allergen, is one of the most common genera found worldwide. Widespread evidence of mold contamination in the school is further illustrated in Figure 1 (fourth floor hallway) and Figure 2 (fourth floor classroom).

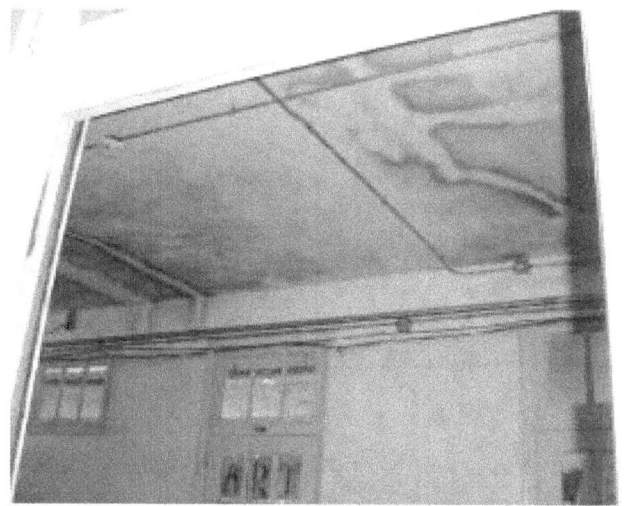

Figure 1. Picture of mold growing along fourth floor hallway cieling at AFSHS

Aureobasidium pullulans, Cladosporium cladosporioides-1, Cladosporium sphaerospermum, and *Eurotium (Asp.) amstelodami* were found in all three MSQPCR air samples with *C. sphaerospermum* being the most prevalent genus (Table C2). The MSQPCR air sample field blank contained no positive hits for fungal spores.

The vacuum dust samples detected 32 of the 35 fungal species tested. The five most prevalent species were *Aspergillus sydowii, Aspergillus unguis, Aureobasidium pullulan, Cladosporium cladosporioides-1*, and *Cladosporium sphaerospermum* (Table C3). The analysis of dust samples by MSQPCR from a national survey of homes conducted by HUD has produced the ERMI for U.S. homes [Vesper et al. 2007]. The ERMI is the result of the analysis for 26 Group 1 mold species

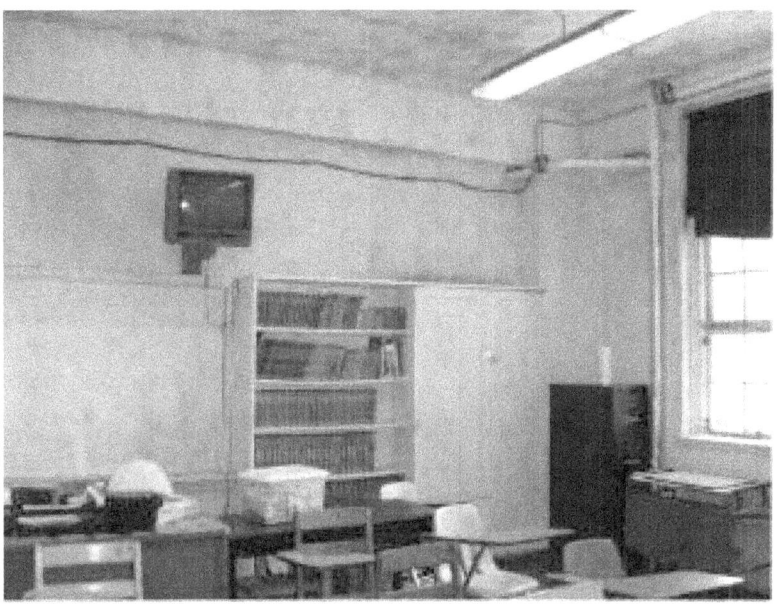

Figure 2. Picture of fourth floor classroom wall and ceiling showing active mold growth at AFSHS

associated with water damage and 10 Group 2 or common species not associated with water damage [Meklin et al. 2004; Vesper et al. 2006]. The ERMI scale ranges from about −10 to 20, lowest to highest [Vesper et al. 2007]. The closer to 20, the greater is the mold burden, indicating likely significant water damage in that environment. The results of the ERMI analysis (Table C3) indicate a high mold burden in AFSHS and that all the dust samples came from highly water-damaged environments.

Lead levels in the peeling paint chips collected in seven rooms ranged from 11 to 1730 µg lead/g total dust (Table C4). The sampling was done to determine whether lead was present in the paint. There are no specific regulations or guidelines for bulk paint samples; however, HUD and U.S. EPA have issued clean-up guidelines for lead on surfaces that can be found in Appendix B.

The culturable air samples for fungi show that *Cladosporium* and *Pencillium* were the most prevalent genera both inside and outside the school (Table C5). *Aspergillus* species were detected in the inside air samples but not in the outside air samples. Air samples from two classrooms with open windows had similar genera and fungal counts to the outside samples.

The spore trap samples showed that *Cladosporium* was the prevalent genus both inside and outside the school with the exception of Room

316, which had *Aspergillus/Pencillum*-like spores as the most prevalent genera (Table C6). The spore counts in the two rooms with closed windows were lower than in the two rooms with open windows and in the outside air sample.

Condensation was observed in classrooms near the top of walls and in the adjacent hallways. The fourth floor had visible evidence of water damage. Room 403 had broken and missing ceiling tiles and holes in the plaster walls. Rooms 407, 408, and 409 had visible water damage on the ceiling and rust on the metal light fixtures. The fourth floor hallway ceiling showed that a large roof leak had been repaired, but the interior damage had not been fixed. The exterior wall on the fourth floor also had a large crack. The moisture readings for May 2005 showed the following: hallway outside Room 208: 10%–12%, interior walls of the third floor stairwell: 30%, exterior walls of the third floor stairwell: 70%–90%, fourth floor exterior wall near the stairwell: about 80%, and fourth floor hallway: 25%–30%. These readings indicated recent water intrusion problems in the third floor stairway and the exterior fourth floor of AFSHS.

Classrooms contained numerous windows, many of which were open during the two site visits in 2005. In April 2005, spot checks for IEQ parameters were made in five classrooms, the teachers' lounge, and the second floor hallway. CO_2 concentrations ranged from 465 ppm to 744 ppm, temperatures ranged from 73.6°F to 78.1°F, and RH levels ranged from 39.8% to 52.4% indoors. These IEQ parameters were within accepted ANSI/ASHRAE guidelines [ANSI/ASHRAE 2004; ANSI/ASHRAE 2007]. In May 2005, spot checks in four classrooms found that CO_2 concentrations ranged from 530 ppm to 576 ppm. When windows are open, the CO_2 concentrations usually reflect the conditions outdoors, not what is happening in the indoor environment. Temperatures ranged from 67.8°F to 79.8°F, and RH levels ranged from 48.3% to 76%. Outside the front door of the school in the morning, the CO_2 level was 422 ppm, the temperature was 90.7°F, and the RH was 49.2%. The May 2005 IEQ measurements for temperature and relative humidity were higher than the ANSI/ASHRAE recommended guidelines [ANSI/ASHRAE 2004; ANSI/ASHRAE 2007]. Additional information on the ANSI/ASHRAE guidelines can be found in Appendix B.

Walnut Hills High School

Eight sticky tape samples were collected at WHHS. No fungal growth was detected in six of the samples. Two of the samples collected in Room 102 showed some evidence of fungal growth – one had a trace of hyphae, and the other showed a few *Aspergillus/Pencillium*-like spores and a trace of hyphae (Table C7). Air samples analyzed with MSQPCR showed low counts for the four inside samples when compared to the outside samples (Table C8). The culturable and spore trap air samples collected inside and outside WHHS were comparable in terms of both counts and genera ranking (Tables C9 and C10).

Rooms 102 and 103, located under a concrete patio, had a history of water leakage. The library had undergone mold remediation several years prior after a leaking roof had been repaired. Some areas of the oldest school building showed evidence that leaks had been repaired but lacked visual evidence of ongoing water intrusion or microbial growth.

In March 2006, IEQ measurements in six classrooms found that CO_2 concentrations ranged from 615 to 1967 ppm, temperatures ranged from 68.9°F to 76.6°F, and RH ranged from 15.7% to 30.8%. Outside the front door of the school, the CO_2 level was 449 to 482 ppm, the temperature was 53.6°F to 59.2°F, and the RH was 49.2%. The rooms with the highest CO_2 concentrations were fully occupied and located in the oldest school building. The elevated CO_2 concentrations indicated a problem with the amount of outdoor air being introduced into the space. Additional information concerning CO_2 concentrations can be found in Appendix B.

DISCUSSION

Some AFSHS employees reported work-related symptoms shown to be associated with occupancy in damp and/or moldy buildings, including upper and lower respiratory symptoms and possibly development of asthma. Twenty AFSHS employees without current, physician-diagnosed asthma met our case definition of work-related asthma, and AFSHS employees who reported current asthma were significantly more likely to report that their asthma was worse at work than were WHHS employees with asthma. Compared to WHHS participants, those at AFSHS had significantly elevated prevalences of constitutional symptoms such as fever, body aches, and unusual tiredness, which, along with cough and shortness of breath, could indicate a history of hypersensitivity pneumonitis.

ERMI scores were high, and epidemiologic studies indicate that higher ERMI values increase the likelihood of asthma/wheeze and rhinitis in children in the home [Vesper et al. 2006; Vesper et al. 2007]. Although the ERMI scale was developed for homes in the United States, finding a very high ERMI value in a school or office would also be strongly suggestive of a water-damaged environment. The dampness and mold in AFSHS were verified by additional environmental sampling including the use of a moisture meter and surface and air samples.

VCS testing is part of a panel of neurobehavioral tests recommended by the Agency for Toxic Substances and Disease Registry for use in community studies of residents exposed to neurotoxins [Amler et al. 1996; Sizemore and Amler 1996]. The adult panel has 12 tests, and the pediatric panel has 15 tests. The Agency for Toxic Substances and Disease Registry selected these tests to assess different aspects of central nervous system functions. These include sensation, motor control, cognition, and affect. The Agency for Toxic Substances and Disease Registry notes that these neurobehavioral tests are for use as nonspecific screening tools that require follow up of positive findings with "appropriate focused tests to characterize more completely any neurotoxic effects that may be present and their relationship to putative exposures" [Amler et al. 1996]. The Agency also states there is no evidence that the tests will identify past exposures to neurotoxins, but they "will detect, without specificity, subtle neurobehavioral changes that may be consequent to many insults" [Amler et al. 1996].

As noted in the introduction, VCS testing has been used in "diagnosing" and monitoring treatment of "biotoxin-related illness" among individuals exposed to water-damaged buildings [Shoemaker and House 2005; Shoemaker and House 2006]. Of particular interest here is that the studies of individuals exposed to water-damaged buildings had several methodologic problems that limit their validity, including nonrepresentative participants, inclusion of persons with specific medical conditions that often present with multiple system symptoms (fibromyalgia and chronic fatigue syndrome), lack of a comparison group, and poor exposure assessment.

We attempted to address some of those issues in this evaluation. We compared VCS scores and symptoms of employees in the damp, moldy school to those of employees in a school without significant dampness or fungal contamination. All employees were asked to participate. Participation was relatively high at both schools, so that not only persons who had significant health issues made up our study population. We conducted a thorough building evaluation at both schools and documented extensive fungal contamination throughout AFSHS, and the lack of significant fungal contamination at WHHS.

Our VCS findings may be due to some factor other than the extensive water damage and mold contamination in AFSHS. We did not examine all possible exposures that may be present in damp buildings, and it is still unclear exactly what exposures in damp buildings are responsible for health effects [WHO 2009]. In addition to mold, dust mites, bacteria, and chemical emissions can be present. We postulated that upper and lower respiratory symptoms and their potential treatment may have led to constitutional and neurobehavioral symptoms and lower VCS scores among these employees. Studies have clearly demonstrated that some persons with allergic rhinitis or asthma complain of fatigue, sleepiness, poor concentration, poor work or school performance, poor sleep, and irritability [Bender 2005; Leander et al. 2009; Williams et al. 2009]. In addition, objective evidence of cognitive impairment (impaired mood, decreased reaction time, attention, and memory) has been demonstrated in persons with allergic rhinitis and asthma [Fitzpatrick et al. 1991; Weersink et al. 1997; Bender 2005]. No studies were located of VCS testing in subjects with allergic diseases such as rhinitis and asthma.

We do not recommend using VCS testing in a clinical setting to diagnose illness in occupants of water-damaged buildings because of its nonspecificity. We were able to detect significant differences in VCS between these two groups of employees, but most employees at AFSHS had normal contrast sensitivity, i.e., that which would be seen in 90% of the population. VCS testing has not been validated as a

DISCUSSION

standalone test for diagnosing neurobehavioral deficits in individuals, but is used by the Agency for Toxic Substances and Disease Registry as part of a panel for assessing populations.

It is possible that the use of a comparison school from a different region of the country could have biased our study. The racial distributions of Cincinnati and New Orleans are very different. In 2000, Cincinnati was 84% white and 13% black; while New Orleans was 55% white and 37% black [CensusScope 2010]. We did not collect information on race or education for our participants because we planned to use another school in the NOPS as our comparison until Hurricane Katrina hit New Orleans. The salaries for teachers in the NOPS District ranged from $25,439 to $41,478 in 2002–2003, while those of Cincinnati Public School teachers ranged from $34,888 to $69,609 in 2003–2004 [US Cities 2009]. This implies a lower socioeconomic status for the employees of AFSHS, which may be associated with poorer health overall and perhaps substandard housing, which may be more prone to leaks and subsequent mold growth. However, a similar proportion of employees at both schools reported mold or moisture problems at home (6%–8%). Lead paint was present in AFSHS. It should have been present in both schools based on the age of the two buildings, but no peeling paint was observed at WHHS, so we did not test for it at WHHS. Lead exposure has been documented to adversely affect VCS. Finally, the cross-sectional nature of our evaluation does not allow for determination of cause-effect relationships.

CONCLUSIONS

We found that a health hazard existed at AFSHS. Employees had significantly higher prevalences of rashes and nasal, lower respiratory, and constitutional symptoms than employees at WHHS. The prevalences of several neurobehavioral symptoms were also significantly higher. VCS values across all spatial frequencies were lower in the employees at AFSHS. Further studies are needed to determine what factors could be responsible for the findings.

RECOMMENDATIONS

Because AFSHS is no longer part of the NOPS district, the following recommendations are offered to the NOPS District to maintain good IEQ and prevent problems for staff. Additional recommendations are provided to address the issues identified for WHHS.

1. Implement an IEQ Management Plan for the NOPS to address IEQ issues. An IEQ manager or administrator with clearly defined responsibilities, authority, and resources should be selected. This individual should have a good understanding of the building's structure and function, and should be able to effectively communicate with occupants. Although no comprehensive regulatory standards specific to IEQ have been established, guidelines have been developed by organizations such as ASHRAE, NIOSH, and the U.S. EPA. An employee representative should be included in the program. The U.S. EPA Indoor Air Quality Tools for Schools program may be helpful for developing and implementing the IEQ management plan. The U.S. EPA has a website specifically for IEQ issues in schools at http://www.epa.gov/iaq/schools/. Information on consultants is available from the AIHA's "Guidelines for Selecting an Indoor Air Quality Consultant".

2. Develop a comprehensive program for the NOPS District to immediately address and fix moisture incursion problems when they occur.

3. Clean up mold contamination when identified in NOPS District buildings using appropriate techniques as outlined in the U.S. EPA document "Mold Remediation in Schools and Commercial Buildings" at http://www.epa.gov/mold/mold_remediation.html and the New York City Department of Health and Mental Hygiene guidelines at http://www.nyc.gov/html/doh/html/epi/moldrpt1.shtml.

4. Reassess the existing preventive maintenance program for the HVAC units in NOPS District buildings to make sure that it meets current needs. Ventilation units in the schools should provide at least the minimum amount of outdoor air according to current ASHRAE guidelines [ANSI/ASHRAE 2007]. Temperature and RH should be measured to determine if current guidelines are being met [ANSI/ASHRAE 2004].

5. Establish a forum, such as a health and safety committee, for all employees to communicate their health concerns to the NOPS District.

6. Evaluate and remediate lead paint in the NOPS District buildings to meet federal and state current guidelines. Additional information on lead paint regulations for the State of Louisiana can be found at http://www.deq.louisiana.gov/portal/tabid/2884/Default.aspx.

7. Encourage employees with health concerns related to their workplace to seek evaluation and care from a physician who is residency trained and/or board certified in occupational medicine and is familiar with the types of exposures employees may have had and their health effects. The Association of Occupational and Environmental Clinics (http://www.aoec.org) and the American College of Occupational and Environmental Medicine (http://www.acoem.org) maintain lists of their members.

8. Evaluate the ventilation systems at WHHS to determine if the amount of outdoor air being provided is in accordance with current ANSI/ASHRAE guidelines [ANSI/ASHRAE 2007].

9. Reseal the patio over the band rooms at WHHS and monitored for leaks routinely. The mold contamination in the band rooms should be remediated.

REFERENCES

Amler RW, Gibertini M, Lybarger JA, Hall A, Kakolewski K, Phifer BL, Olsen KL [1996]. Selective approaches to basic neurobehavioral testing of children in environmental health studies. Neurotoxicol Teratol 18(4):429–434.

ANSI/ASHRAE [2004]. Thermal environmental conditions for human occupancy. American National Standards Institute/ASHRAE standard 55-2004. Atlanta, GA: American Society for Heating, Refrigerating, and Air-Conditioning Engineers, Inc.

ANSI/ASHRAE [2007]. Ventilation for acceptable indoor air quality. American National Standards Institute/ASHRAE standard 62.1-2007. Atlanta, GA: American Society of Heating, Refrigerating, and Air-Conditioning Engineers, Inc.

Bartgis J, Lefler EK, Hartung CM, Thomas DG [2009]. Contrast sensitivity in children with and without attention deficit hyperactivity disorder symptoms. Dev Neuropsychol 34(6):663–682.

Bender BG [2005]. Cognitive effects of allergic rhinitis and its treatment. Immunol Allergy Clin N Am 25(2):301–312.

Boeckelmann I, Pfister EA [2003]. Influence of occupational exposure to organic solvent mixtures on contrast sensitivity in printers. J Occup Environ Med 45(1):25–33.

Broadwell DK, Darcey DJ, Hudnell HK, Otto DA, Boyes WK [1995]. Work-site clinical and neurobehavioral assessment of solvent-exposed microelectronics workers. Am J Indust Med 27(5):677–698.

Bubl E, Van Elst LT, Gondan M, Ebert D, Greenlee MW [2009]. Vision in depressive disorder. World J Biol Psychiatry 10(4):377–384.

CensusScope [http://www.censusscope.org/us/metro_rank_race_blackafricanamerican.html]. Date accessed: August 2010.

Fitzpatrick MF, Engleman H, Whyte KF, Deary IJ, Shapiro CM, Douglas NJ [1991]. Morbidity in nocturnal asthma: sleep quality and daytime cognitive performance. Thorax 46(8):569–573.

Frenette B, Mergler D, Bowler R [1991]. Contrast sensitivity loss in a group of former microelectronics workers with normal visual acuity. Optom Vis Sci 68(7):556–560.

References
(continued)

Ginsburg AP [1993]. Functional Acuity Contrast Test F A.C.T.® Instructions for use. Chicago, IL: Stereo Optical Company, Inc.

Gong Y, Kishi R, Kasai S, Katakura Y, Fujiwara K, Umemura T, Kondo T, Sato T, Sata F, Tsukishima E, Tozaki S, Kawai T, Miyama Y [2003]. Visual dysfunction in workers exposed to a mixture of organic solvents. Neurotoxicology 24(4–5):703–710.

Haugland RA, Brinkman NE, Vesper SJ [2002]. Evaluation of rapid DNA extraction methods for the quantitative detection of fungal cells using real time PCR analysis. J Microbiol Meth 50(3):319–323.

Hitchcock EM, Dick RB, Krieg EF [2003]. Visual contrast sensitivity testing: a comparison of two F A.C.T. test types. Neurotoxicol Teratol 26(2):271–277.

Leander M, Cronqvist A, Janson C, Uddenfeldt M, Rask-Andersen A. [2009]. Non-respiratory symptoms and well-being in asthmatics from a general population sample. J Asthma 46(6):552–559.

Meklin T, Haugland RA, Reponen T, Varma M, Lummus Z, Bernstein D, Wymer L J, Vesper S J [2004]. Quantitative PCR analysis of house dust can reveal abnormal mold conditions. J Environ Monitor 6(7):615–20.

Nomura H, Ando F, Niino N, Shimokata H, Miyake Y [2003]. Age-related change in contrast sensitivity among Japanese adults. Jpn J Ophthalmol 47(3):299–303.

Pearson P, Timney B [1999]. Alcohol does not affect visual contrast gain mechanisms. Vis Neurosci 16(4):675–80.

Schreiber JS, Hudnell HK, Geller AM, House DE, Aldous KM, Force MS, Langguth K, Prohonic EJ, Parker JC [2002]. Apartment residents' and day care workers' exposure to tetrachloroethylene and deficits in visual contrast sensitivity. Environ Health Perspect 110(7):655–664.

Shoemaker RC, House DE [2005]. A time-series study of sick building syndrome: chronic, biotoxin-associated illness from exposure to water-damaged buildings. Neurotoxicol Teratol 27(1):29–46.

Shoemaker RC, House DE [2006]. Sick building syndrome and exposure to water-damaged buildings: time series study, clinical trial and mechanisms. Neurotoxicol Teratol 28(5):573–588.

REFERENCES
(CONTINUED)

Sizemore OJ, Amler RW [1996]. Characteristics of ATSDR's adult and pediatric environmental neurobehavioral test batteries. Neurotoxicology 17(1):229–236.

US Cities [2009]. [www.city-data.com/us-cities/The-South/New-Orleans-Education-and-Research.html]. Date accessed: August 2010.

Vesper SJ, McKinstry C, Yang C, Haugland RA, Kercsmar CM, Yike I, Schluchter MD, Kirchner HL, Sobolewski J, Allan TM, Dearborn DG [2006]. Specific molds associated with asthma. J Occup Environ Med 48(8):852–858.

Vesper S, McKinstry C, Haugland R, Wymer L, Bradham K, Ashley P, Cox D, Dewalt G, Friedman W [2007]. Development of an environmental relative moldiness index for US homes. J Occup Environ Med 49(8):829–833.

Weersink EJ, van Zomeren EH, Koëter GH, Postma DS [1997]. Treatment of nocturnal airway obstruction improves daytime cognitive performance in asthmatics. Am J Respir Crit Care Med. 156(4 Pt 1):1144–1150.

Williams SA, Wagner S, Kannan H, Bolge SC [2009]. The association between asthma control and health care utilization, work productivity loss, and health-related quality of life. J Occup Environ Med 51(7):780–785.

World Health Organization [2009]. WHO guidelines for indoor air quality: dampness and mould. WHO Regional Office for Europe.

Visual Contrast Sensitivity

Contrast sensitivity testing was conducted with the F.A.C.T. handheld chart [Ginsburg 1993]. This instrument consists of a calibrated rod with a card holder at one end and cheek pads at the other end that are held tightly against the face to maintain a constant viewing distance between the eyes and the test card (Figure 3).

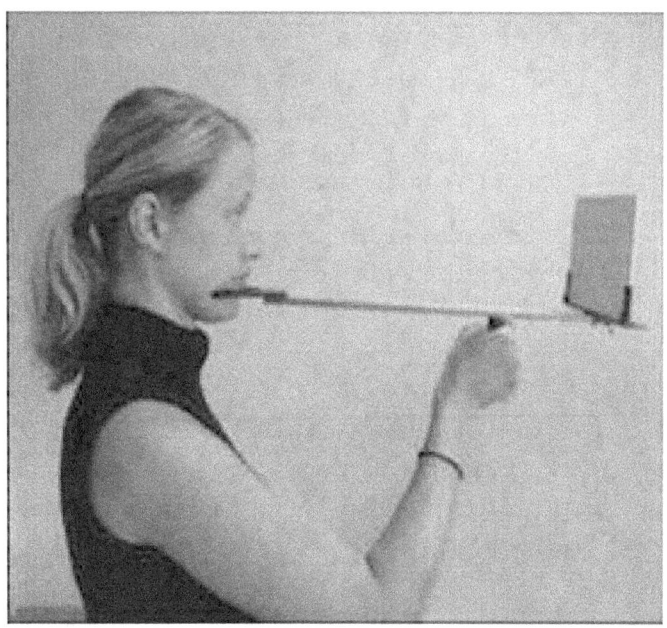

Figure 3: Visual contrast sensitivity test using F.A.C.T. chart.

VCS testing has been used to document subclinical neurobehavioral effects in persons exposed to neurotoxicants and has recently been reported to be affected by exposure to water-damaged buildings. VCS tests are considered superior to visual acuity tests for detecting visual loss. Visual acuity tests (similar to the tests done by optometrists when ordering eyeglasses) generally detect refractive disorders, whereas VCS tests may detect visual changes due to chemical exposures even though visual acuity is normal (e.g., 20/20) [Regan 1989]. VCS can be affected by a number of factors including age, hypertension, diabetes, head injury, alcohol consumption; and various eye conditions such as cataract, glaucoma, LASIK and other eye surgery [Atkin et al. 1979; Sokol et al. 1985; Trick et al. 1988; Roquelaure et al. 1995; Pearson and Timney 1998; Hammond et al. 2004; Shamshinova et al. 2007].

The F.A.C.T. sine-wave grating chart tests five spatial frequencies (1.5, 3, 6, 12, 18 cycles per degree) and nine levels of contrast.

Cycles per degree refers to the number of alternating light and dark bands within one degree of visual angle. Contrast refers to the difference in intensity (expressed as a percent) between the light and dark bands, with white to black having a 100% contrast. The last grating seen for each spatial frequency row, assessed by a correct reporting of the orientation of the grating (right, up, or left), is plotted on a contrast sensitivity curve. Test results produce a visuogram that indicates sensitivity at each of the five spatial frequencies tested. Because high levels of visual sensitivity for spatial form are associated with low contrast thresholds, a reciprocal measure (1/threshold), termed the contrast sensitivity score, is computed. Measures of visual contrast sensitivity, rather than measures of refractory visual acuity, have been presented as better appraisals of visual dysfunction resulting from chemical exposures. However, if visual acuity is poor, then performance on the F.A.C.T. will also be poor. Therefore, we also measured visual acuity with a handheld Snellen chart. Results from persons with visual acuity of 20/50 or less were removed from further analysis.

The tests were conducted monocularly and binocularly under standard daylight illumination in the library of each school. A light meter was used to ensure that ambient illumination met the requirements specified for the F.A.C.T. handheld chart (between 68 and 239 candelas per square meter). Participants who used corrective lenses were asked to wear them during testing. Using a preprinted recording form, the test results indicate where the subject being tested falls in the range of average performance for 90% of the population [Ginsburg 1993].

Environmental Sampling

During the first site visit at AFSHS on April 18–19, 2005, 14 sticky tape samples for microscopic fungal analysis were collected throughout the school. Five vacuum dust samples were collected using a filter "sock" with a HEPA vacuum in Rooms 317, 321, 322, 400, and 426. Three air samples were collected in Room 213, Room 416, and the teachers' lounge with an SKC Inhalable Button™ Sampler (SKC Inc., Eighty Four, Pennsylvania) with a 2.0-µm pore size polycarbonate filter at a flow rate of 3.5 Lpm. These eight samples were analyzed via a DNA-based method called MSQPCR [Haugland et al. 2002]. MSQPCR identifies 36 species of fungi commonly associated with water-damaged indoor environments using established procedures for preparing conidial suspensions from fungal cultures, extracting DNA, and performing MSQPCR analyses [Haugland et al. 2002; Brinkman et al. 2003; Haugland et al. 2004]. All primer and probe sequences, as well as known species comprising the assay groups, were published at http://www.epa.gov/microbes/moldtech.htm. A TRAMEX Moisture Encounter meter (Tramex Ltd., Littleton, Colorado) was used to qualitatively assess the interior wall moisture levels. To address requestors' concerns over the potential for lead exposures from peeling paint, paint samples were collected in six rooms in April 2005 and one room in May 2005 and analyzed for lead according to NIOSH Method 7300 using inductively coupled plasma atomic emission spectrometry [NIOSH 2010].

During the second site visit to AFSHS, a more detailed environmental evaluation was conducted. Air sampling using Andersen N-6 samplers (Thermo Electron Corporation, Waltham, Massachusetts) with MEA agar plates at a flow rate of 28.3 Lpm was performed in four classrooms (Rooms 205, 316, 420, and 427) and one outdoor location. A sampling time of 5 minutes was used. All N-6 samples were collected in triplicate. All sampling pumps were pre- and post-calibrated with a DryCal (Bios International Corporation, Butler, New Jersey).

Spore trap samples were collected with Air-o-Cell® samplers (Zefon International, Inc , Ocala, Florida) at a flow rate of 15 Lpm in the same sampling locations. A sampling time of 5 minutes was used. All spore trap samples were collected in triplicate. Measurements of CO_2, temperature, and RH were made throughout the workday using TSI Q-Trak™ Indoor Air Quality monitors (TSI Incorporated, Shoreview, Minnesota). Two additional sticky tape samples were collected for microscopic fungal analysis. One additional paint sample was collected and analyzed for lead using NIOSH Method 7300 [NIOSH 2010].

A similar environmental protocol was used for the WHHS evaluation, except for lead paint sampling. Eight sticky tape samples were collected and submitted for microscopic fungal analysis. The sampled areas were Band Room 102 (three samples), Band Room 103 (two samples), library (two samples), and Room 333 (one sample). Air sampling using Andersen N-6 samplers with MEA agar plates at a flow rate of 28.3 Lpm was performed in four classrooms and the library (Rooms 102, 260, 333, and 334) and one outdoor location. A sampling time of 5 minutes was used. All N-6 samples were collected in triplicate. All sampling pumps were pre- and post-calibrated with a DryCal. Area air samples were collected in the same locations using a 0.3 µm pore-size 37-millimeter polytetrafluoroethylene filter at a flow rate of 2 Lpm. The six area air samples were analyzed for fungal species via MSQPCR.

Spore trap samples were collected with Air-o-Cell samplers at a flow rate of 15 Lpm in the same sampling locations. A sampling time of 5 minutes was used, and all spore trap samples were collected in triplicate. Measurements of CO_2, temperature, and RH were made throughout the workday using TSI Q-Trak Indoor Air Quality monitors.

Statistical Analysis

SAS Version 9.1.3 software (SAS Institute, Cary, North Carolina) and StatXact Version 6 software (Cytel Software Corporation, Cambridge, Massachusetts) were used for the statistical analyses. Results with P values ≤ 0.05 were considered statistically significant. Chi square or Fisher's exact tests were used to compare the prevalence of symptoms, certain demographic characteristics, and percent of abnormal VCS scores between schools. To examine the relationship between work-related symptoms and VCS values, we combined the symptoms into the following symptom complexes: upper respiratory (sinus problems, dry or irritated eyes, nosebleeds, sore or dry throat, frequent sneezing, stuffy nose, or runny nose); lower respiratory (cough, wheezing or whistling in the chest, chest tightness, or unusual shortness of breath); and neurobehavioral (difficulty concentrating, trouble remembering things, confusion or disorientation, irritability, depression, or change in sleep patterns). The Wilcoxon two-sample test was used to compare alcohol intake and VCS values between schools, and to examine the relationship between symptom complexes and VCS values. Mold concentration data having a minimum detection limit of 1 cell per milligram dust were treated as left-censored data with appropriate statistical methods applied [Helsel 2005]. Procedurally, nondetections were set at half the minimum detection limit, and given equal and lowest rank for nonparametric rank-based analyses [Helsel 2005].

References

Atkin A, Bodis-Wollner I, Wolkstein M, Moss A, Podos SM [1979]. Abnormalities in central contrast sensitivity in glaucoma. Am J Ophthalmol 88(2):205–211.

Brinkman NE, Haugland RA, Wymer LJ, Byappanahalli M, Whitman RL, Vesper SJ [2003]. Evaluation of a rapid, quantitative real-time PCR method for cellular enumeration of pathogenic *Candida* species in water. Appl Environ Microbiol 69(3):1775–1782.

Ginsburg AP [1993]. Functional Acuity Contrast Test F A.C.T.® Instructions for use. Chicago, IL: Stereo Optical Company, Inc.

Hammond SD Jr, Puri AK, Ambati BK [2004]. Quality of vision and patient satisfaction after LASIK. Curr Opin Ophthalmol 15(4):328–332.

Haugland RA, Brinkman NE, Vesper SJ [2002]. Evaluation of rapid DNA extraction methods for the quantitative detection of fungal cells using real time PCR analysis. J Microbiol Meth 50(3):319–323.

Haugland RA, Varma M, Wymer LJ, Vesper SJ [2004]. Quantitative PCR of selected *Aspergillus*, *Penicillium* and *Paecilomyces* species. Sys Appl Microbiol 27(2):198–210.

Helsel DR [2005]. Nondetects and data analysis, statistics for censored environmental data. Wiley and Sons Inc. Hoboken, NJ.

NIOSH [2010]. NIOSH manual of analytical methods (NMAM®). 4th ed. Schlecht PC, O'Connor PF, eds. Cincinnati, OH: U.S. Department of Health and Human Services, Public Health Service, Centers for Disease Control and Prevention, National Institute for Occupational Safety and Health, DHHS (NIOSH) Publication 94–113 (August, 1994); 1st Supplement Publication 96–135, 2nd Supplement Publication 98–119; 3rd Supplement 2003–154. [http://www.cdc.gov/niosh/nmam/]. Date accessed: August 2010.

Pearson P, Timney B [1998]. Effects of moderate blood alcohol concentrations on spatial and temporal contrast sensitivity. J Stud Alcohol 59(2):163–173.

Regan D [1989]. Human brain electrophysiology. New York: Elsevier, p. 672.

Roquelaure Y, Gargasson LE, Kupper S, Girre C, Hispard E, Dally S [1995]. Alcohol consumption and visual contrast sensitivity. Alcohol Alcohol 30(5):681–685.

Shamshinova AM, Arakelian MA, Rogova SIu, Adasheve TV, Silakova OL [2007]. Classification of the forms of hypertensive retinopathy on the basis of estimation of the bioelectrical retinal potential and contrast sensitivity. Vestn Oftalmol 123(1):24–28.

Sokol S, Moskowitz A, Skarf B, Evans R, Molitch M, Senior B [1985]. Contrast sensitivity in diabetics with and without background retinopathy. Arch Ophthalmol 103(1):51–54.

Trick GL, Burde RM, Gordon MO, Santiago JV, Kilo C [1988]. The relationship between hue discrimination and contrast sensitivity deficits in patients with diabetes mellitus. Ophthalmology 95(5):693–698.

Microbial Contamination

Exposure to microbes is not unique to the indoor environment. No environment, indoors or out, is completely free from microbes, not even a surgical operating room. Remediation of microbial contamination may improve IEQ conditions even though a specific cause-effect relationship is not determined. NIOSH investigators routinely recommend the remediation of observed microbial contamination and the correction of situations that are favorable for microbial growth and bioaerosol dissemination.

Mold

The types and severity of symptoms related to exposure to mold in the indoor environment depend in part on the extent of the mold present, the extent of the individual's exposure, and the susceptibility of the individual (for example, whether he or she has preexisting allergies or asthma). In general, excessive exposure to fungi may produce health problems by several primary mechanisms, including allergy or hypersensitivity, infection, and toxic effects. Additionally, molds produce a variety of VOCs, the most common of which is ethanol, that have been postulated to cause upper airway irritation. However, as discussed above, potential irritant effects of VOCs from exposure to mold in the indoor environment are not well understood. Evidence also shows that exposure to fungal fragments that can contain allergens, toxins, and $(1{\rightarrow}3){-}\beta{-}D{-}$glucan may occur [Górney et al. 2002; Brasel et al. 2005; Reponen et al. 2006].

Allergic responses are the most common type of health problem associated with exposure to molds. These health problems may include sneezing; itching of the nose, eyes, mouth, or throat; nasal stuffiness and runny nose; and red, itchy eyes. Repeated or single exposure to mold or mold spores may cause previously nonsensitized individuals to become sensitized. Molds can trigger asthma symptoms (shortness of breath, wheezing, cough) in persons who are allergic to mold. In the 2004 report, "Damp Indoor Spaces and Health," the IOM found sufficient evidence of an association between mold or dampness indoors and nasal and throat symptoms, asthma symptoms in sensitized asthmatics, wheeze, cough, and hypersensitivity pneumonitis in susceptible persons [IOM 2004]. The IOM found limited or suggestive evidence of an association between lower respiratory illness in healthy children and damp indoor spaces. Evidence was inadequate or insufficient to determine whether an association exists between dyspnea, airflow obstruction in healthy persons, mucous membrane irritation, skin symptoms, chronic obstructive pulmonary disease, asthma development, inhalation fevers in nonoccupational settings, fatigue, cancer, reproductive effects, neuropsychiatric effects, lower respiratory illness in healthy adults, gastrointestinal problems, rheumatologic or immune problems, or acute idiopathic pulmonary hemorrhage in infants. No health conditions met the level of evidence for causation. In 2009, WHO published guidelines for protection of public health from mold and other exposures in damp buildings [WHO 2009]. Based on its review of the scientific literature for this report, the WHO concluded that there was sufficient epidemiologic evidence that occupants of damp buildings are at risk of developing upper and lower respiratory tract symptoms (including cough, wheeze, and dyspnea), respiratory infections, asthma, and exacerbation of asthma. The WHO also concluded that limited evidence suggests an association between bronchitis and allergic rhinitis and damp buildings. It noted clinical evidence that exposure to mold and other microbial agents in damp buildings is associated with hypersensitivity pneumonitis.

People with weakened immune systems (immune-compromised or immune-suppressed individuals) may be more vulnerable to infections by molds. For example, *Aspergillus fumigatus* is a fungal species that has been found almost everywhere on every conceivable type of substrate. It has been known to infect the lungs of immune-compromised individuals after inhalation of the airborne spores [Wald and Stave 1994; Brandt et al. 2006]. Healthy individuals are usually not vulnerable to infections from airborne mold exposure.

No exposure guidelines for mold in air exist, so it is not possible to distinguish between "safe" and "unsafe" levels of exposure. Nevertheless, the potential for health problems is an important reason to prevent indoor mold growth and to remediate any indoor mold contamination. Moisture intrusion, along with nutrient sources such as building materials or furnishings, allows mold to grow indoors, so it is important to keep the building interior and furnishings dry. NIOSH concurs with the U.S. EPA's recommendations to remedy mold contamination in indoor environments (http://www.epa.gov/iaq/molds/mold_remediation.html) [Redd SC 2002; U.S. EPA 2001a]. Additional information on health effects and mold remediation can be found in the CDC document "Mold Prevention Strategies and Possible Health Effects in the Aftermath of Hurricanes and Major Floods" at http://www.cdc.gov/mmwr/preview/mmwrhtml/rr5508a1.htm.

No standards specific to the nonindustrial indoor environment exist. Measurement of indoor environmental contaminants has seldom proved helpful in determining the cause of symptoms except where there are unusual sources, or a proven relationship between specific exposures and disease. With few exceptions, concentrations of frequently measured chemical substances in the indoor work environment fall well below the recommended OELs published by NIOSH [NIOSH 2005], ACGIH [ACGIH 2010], and AIHA [AIHA 2010], and the mandatory PELs set by OSHA [29 CFR 1910 (general industry)]. ANSI/ASHRAE has published recommended building ventilation and thermal comfort guidelines [ANSI/ASHRAE 2004; ANSI/ASHRAE 2007]. The ACGIH and AIHA have also developed a manual of guidelines for approaching investigations of building-related symptoms that might be caused by airborne living organisms or their effluents [ACGIH 1999; AIHA 2008]. Other resources that provide guidance for establishing acceptable IEQ are available through U.S. EPA at http://www.epa.gov/iaq, especially the U.S. EPA Indoor Air Quality Tools for Schools (http://www.epa.gov/iaq/schools/), and the joint U.S. EPA/NIOSH document, *Building Air Quality, A Guide for Building Owners and Facility Managers* (http://www.epa.gov/iaq/largebldgs/baqtoc.html).

Heating, Ventilating, and Air-Conditioning

One of the most common deficiencies in the indoor environment is the improper operation and maintenance of ventilation systems and other building components [Rosenstock 1996]. NIOSH investigators have found correcting HVAC problems often reduces reported symptoms. Most studies of ventilation rates and building occupant symptoms have shown that rates below 10 Ls^{-1}/person (which equates to 20 cubic feet per minute per person) are associated with one or more health symptoms [Seppanen et al 1999]. Moreover, higher ventilation rates, from 10 Ls^{-1}/person up to 20 Ls^{-1}/person, have been associated with further significant decreases in the prevalence of symptoms [Seppanen et al. 1999]. Thus, improved HVAC operation and maintenance, higher ventilation rates, and comfortable temperature and RH can all potentially serve to improve symptoms without ever identifying any specific cause-effect relationships. When conducting an IEQ evaluation, NIOSH investigators often measure ventilation and comfort indicators, such as CO_2, temperature, and RH to provide information relative to the functioning and control of HVAC systems.

Carbon Dioxide

CO_2 is a normal constituent of exhaled breath and is not considered a building air pollutant. It can be used as an indicator of whether sufficient quantities of outdoor air are being introduced into an occupied space for acceptable odor control. However, CO_2 is not an effective indicator of ventilation adequacy if the ventilated area is not occupied at its usual occupant density at the time the CO_2 is measured. ASHRAE notes in an informative appendix to standard 62.1 that indoor CO_2 concentrations no greater than 700 ppm above outdoor CO_2 concentrations will satisfy a substantial majority (about 80%) of visitors with regard to odor from sedentary building occupants (body odor) [ANSI/ASHRAE 2007]. Elevated CO_2 concentrations suggest that other indoor contaminants may also be increased. If CO_2 concentrations are elevated, the amount of outdoor air introduced into the ventilated space may need to be increased. When CO_2 concentrations are used as an indicator to determine outdoor air requirements, ventilation system designs that rely on duct-mounted CO_2 sensors should have some form of ventilation efficiency documentation that relates concentration values observed at the duct location with those observed within the breathing zone of the occupied space.

Temperature and Relative Humidity

Temperature and RH measurements are often collected as part of an IEQ evaluation because these parameters affect the perception of comfort in an indoor environment. The perception of thermal comfort is related to one's metabolic heat production, the transfer of heat to the environment, physiological adjustments, and body temperature [NIOSH 1986]. Heat transfer from the body to the environment is influenced by factors such as temperature, humidity, air movement, personal activities, and clothing. The ANSI/ASHRAE Standard 55-2004: *Thermal Environmental Conditions for Human Occupancy*, specifies conditions in which 80% or more of the occupants would be expected to find the environment thermally acceptable [ANSI/ASHRAE 2004]. Assuming slow air movement and 50% RH, the operative temperatures recommended by ANSI/ASHRAE range from 68.5°F to 76°F in the winter and from 75°F to 80.5°F in the summer. The difference between the two is largely due to seasonal clothing selection. ANSI/ASHRAE also recommends that RH be maintained at or below 65% [ANSI/ASHRAE 2007]. Excessive humidity can promote the excessive growth of microorganisms and dust mites.

Lead in Surface Dust and Soil

Lead is ubiquitous in U.S. urban environments because of the widespread use of lead compounds in industry, gasoline, and paints during the past century. Occupational exposure to lead occurs via inhalation of dust and fume and via ingestion through contact with lead-contaminated hands, food, cigarettes, and clothing. Absorbed lead accumulates in the body in the soft tissues and bones [ATSDR 1990]. Lead is stored in bones for decades, and may cause health effects long after exposure as it is slowly released in the body.

Lead-contaminated surface dust represents a potential source of lead exposure, particularly for young children. This may occur either by direct hand-to-mouth contact, or indirectly from hand-to-mouth contact with contaminated clothing, cigarettes, or food. Previous studies have found a significant correlation between resident children's BLLs and house dust lead levels [Farfel and Chisholm 1990].

In the workplace, generally there is little or no correlation between surface lead levels and employee exposures because ingestion exposures are highly dependent on personal hygiene practices and available facilities for maintaining personal hygiene. No current federal standard provides an exposure limit for lead contamination of surfaces in the workplace. The OSHA lead standard requires maintaining all surfaces as free as practicable of accumulations of lead. Additionally, OSHA has stated in its Compliance Directive CPL 02-02-058-29 CFR 1926.62, Lead Exposure In Construction; Interim Final Rule: Inspection and Compliance Procedures (12/13/1993), that it recommends the use of HUD's recommended level for acceptable decontamination of 200 $\mu g/ft^2$ for floors in evaluating cleanliness of change areas, storage facilities, and lunchrooms/eating areas and would not expect that surfaces should be any cleaner than this level [OSHA 1993].

The U.S. EPA currently recommends meeting the following clearance levels for surface lead loading after residential lead abatement or interim control activities: floors, 40 $\mu g/ft^2$; interior window sills, 250 $\mu g/ft^2$; window troughs, 400 $\mu g/ft^2$ [U.S. EPA 2001b]. These levels have been established as achievable through lead abatement and interim control activities. They are not based on projected health effects associated with specific surface dust levels. The Louisiana Department of Environmental Quality has a website containing state specific information about lead-based paint at http://www.deq.louisiana.gov/portal/tabid/2884/Default.aspx.

References

ACGIH [1999]. Bioaerosols: assessment and control. Cincinnati, OH: American Conference of Governmental Industrial Hygienists.

ACGIH [2010]. 2010 TLVs® and BEIs®: threshold limit values for chemical substances and physical agents and biological exposure indices. Cincinnati, OH: American Conference of Governmental Industrial Hygienists.

AIHA [2008]. Recognition, evaluation, and control of indoor mold. Prezant B, Weekes DM, Miller JD eds. Fairfax, VA: American Industrial Hygiene Association.

AIHA [2010]. 2010 Emergency response planning guidelines (ERPG) & workplace environmental exposure levels (WEEL) handbook. Fairfax, VA: American Industrial Hygiene Association.

ANSI/ASHRAE [2004]. Thermal environmental conditions for human occupancy. American National Standards Institute/ASHRAE standard 55-2004. Atlanta, GA: American Society for Heating, Refrigerating, and Air-Conditioning Engineers, Inc.

ANSI/ASHRAE [2007]. Ventilation for acceptable indoor air quality. American National Standards Institute/ASHRAE standard 62.1-2007. Atlanta, GA: American Society of Heating, Refrigerating, and Air-Conditioning Engineers, Inc.

ATSDR [1990]. Toxicological profile for lead. Atlanta, GA: U.S. Department of Health and Human Services, Agency for Toxic Substances and Disease Registry. DHHS (ATSDR) Publication No. TP–88/17.

Brandt M, Brown C, Burkhart J, Burton N, Cox-Ganser J, Damon S, Falk H, Fridkin S, Garbe P, McGeehin M, Morgan J, Page E, Rao C, Redd S, Sinks T, Trout D, Wallingford K, Warnock D, Weissman D [2006]. Mold prevention strategies and possible health effects in the aftermath of hurricanes and major floods. MMWR 55(RR-8):1–27.

Brasel TL, Martin JM, Carriker CG, Wilson SC, Straus DC [2005]. Detection of airborne *Stachybotrys chartarum* macrocyclic trichothecene mycotoxins in the indoor environment. Appl Environ Microbiol 71(11):7376–7388.

CFR. Code of Federal Regulations. Washington, DC: U.S. Government Printing Office, Office of the Federal Register.

Farfel MR, Chisholm JJ [1990]. Health and environmental outcomes of traditional and modified practices for abatement of residential lead–based paint. Am J Pub Health 80(10):1240–1245.

Górny RL, Reponen T, Willeke K, Schmechel D, Robine E, Boissier M, Grinshpun SA [2002]. Fungal fragments as indoor air biocontaminants. Appl Environ Microbiol 68(7):3522–3531.

IOM [2004]. Human health effects associated with damp indoor environments. In: Damp indoor spaces and health. Washington, DC: Institute of Medicine, National Academy Press, pp. 183–269.

NIOSH [1986]. Criteria for a recommended standard: occupational exposure to hot environments, revised criteria. Cincinnati, OH: U.S. Department of Health and Human Services, Centers for Disease Control, National Institute for Occupational Safety and Health, DHHS (NIOSH) Publication No. 86-13.

NIOSH [2005]. NIOSH pocket guide to chemical hazards. Cincinnati, OH: U.S. Department of Health and Human Services, Centers for Disease Control and Prevention, National Institute for Occupational Safety and Health, DHHS (NIOSH) Publication No. 2005-149. [http://www.cdc.gov/niosh/npg/]. Date accessed: August 2010.

OSHA [1993]. Occupational Safety and Health Administration Instruction CPL 02-02-058-29 CFR 1926.62, Lead Exposure in Construction; Interim Final Rule: Inspection and Compliance Procedures (12/13/1993).

Redd SC [2002]. State of the science on molds and human health. Statement for the Record Before the Subcommittee on Oversight and Investigations and Housing and Community Opportunity, Committee on Financial Services, United States House of Representatives. Atlanta, GA: U.S. Department of Health and Human Services, Centers for Disease Control and Prevention.

Reponen T, Seo S-C, Iossifova Y, Adhikari A, Grinshpun SA [2006]. New field-compatible method for collection and analysis of β-glucan in fungal fragments. Abstracts of the International Aerosol Conference, St. Paul, Minnesota, p. 955.

Rosenstock L [1996]. NIOSH Testimony to the U.S. Department of Labor on indoor air quality. Applied Occupational and Environmental Hygiene 11(12):1365-1370.

Seppanen OA, Fisk WJ, Mendell MJ [1999]. Association of ventilation rates and CO_2 concentrations with health and other responses in commercial and institutional buildings. Indoor Air 9(4):226-252.

U.S. EPA [2001a]. Mold remediation in schools and commercial buildings. Washington, DC: United States Environmental Protection Agency, Office of Air and Radiation, Indoor Environments Division. EPA Publication No. 402-K-01-001.

U.S. EPA [2001b]. Lead; identification of dangerous levels of lead. Washington, DC: United States Environmental Protection Agency. 40 CFR Part 745 [http://www.epa.gov/fedrgstr/EPA-TOX/2001/January/Day-05/t84.pdf]. Date accessed: August 2010.

Wald P, Stave G [1994]. Fungi. In: Physical and biological hazards of the workplace. New York: Van Nostrand Reinhold, p. 394.

WHO [2009]. WHO guidelines for indoor air quality: dampness and mould. Geneva, Switzerland: World Health Organization. [http://www.euro.who.int/document/e92645.pdf]. Date accessed: August 2010.

Table C1. Microscopic sticky tape sample results for AFSHS

Sample location	Genera	Amount of growth*
	April 19, 2005	
2nd floor hallway across from teachers' lounge	*Cladosporium* spores, hyphae, conidiophores	Numerous
Room 217 under window sill – water-damaged	None	
Room 213 wall with dark pattern near door	*Cladosporium* spores, hyphae, conidiophores	Numerous
Room 213 – next to window by teacher's desk	*Cladosporium* spores, hyphae, conidiophores	Numerous
3rd floor hallway across from Room 313	*Cladosporium* spores, hyphae, conidiophores	Numerous
3rd floor hallway across from Room 317	*Cladosporium* spores, hyphae, conidiophores	Numerous
Room 313 – wall over chalkboard	*Cladosporium* spores, hyphae, conidiophores	Massive
4th floor hallway across from Room 400	*Cladosporium* spores, hyphae, conidiophores	Massive
Room 416 – wall over chalkboard	*Cladosporium* spores, hyphae, conidiophores	Many
4th floor hallway black pattern on ceiling	*Cladosporium* spores, hyphae, conidiophores	Massive
3rd floor hallway outside of library	*Cladosporium* spores, hyphae, conidiophores	Numerous
3rd floor faculty women's restroom	*Cladosporium* spores, hyphae, conidiophores	Massive
Room 312A ceiling	*Cladosporium* spores, hyphae, conidiophores	Massive
Room 316 wall	*Cladosporium* spores, hyphae, conidiophores	Massive
	May 24, 2005	
2nd floor hallway by Room 208	*Cladosporium* spores, hyphae, conidiophores	Numerous
Room 205 wall	*Cladosporium* spores, hyphae, conidiophores	Massive

*Massive>numerous>many>a few>trace

Table C2. Fungal spore equivalents in air identified by MSQPCR in the AFSHS on April 19, 2005

Sample locations	2nd Floor Teachers' Lounge	Room 213	Room 416
Sampling time	9:34 a.m. – 3:42 p.m.	9:42 a.m. – 3:34 p.m.	9:46 a.m. – 3:37 p.m.
Fungal ID (SE/m^3)*			
Aspergillus fumigatus	0	0	10
Aspergillus niger	5	4	0
Aspergillus penicillioides	54	21	0
Aspergillus unguis	2	0	0
Aspergillus versicolor	29	0	0
Aureobasidium pullulans	2	2	5
Cladosporium cladosporioides-1	212	757	426
Cladosporium cladosporioides-2	8	0	1
Cladosporium sphaerospermum	52	29	33
Epicoccum nigrum	0	0	41
Eurotium (Asp.) amstelodami	89	1	4
Mucor amphibiorum group	1	0	0
Penicillium brevicompactum	6	0	0
Penicillium crustosum (group 2)	0	0	19211
Penicillium variabile	0	0	3
Rhizopus stolonifer	0	1	0
Scopulariopsis brevicaulis/fusca	0	0	154
Wallemia sebi	0	3	147

*Spore equivalent per cubic meter of air

Table C3. Fungal spore equivalents in dust using MSQPCR and ERMI analysis AFSHS on April 19, 2005

Fungal species Group 1	Room 321 wall by teacher's desk	Room 317 by teacher's desk	Room 426 Top of filing cabinet	Room 322 Choir Room chairs	Room 400 window sill
Aspergillus flavus	6	5	31	7	1
Aspergillus fumigatus	14	3	94	13	7
Aspergillus niger	9	2	16	7	22
Aspergillus ochraceus	1	1	1	1	1
Aspergillus penicillioides	743	211	351	47	55
Aspergillus restrictus	1	1	63	1	1
Aspergillus sclerotiorum	76	38	196	104	1
Aspergillus sydowii	1174	214	67	1	113
Aspergillus unguis	4504	237	375	52	2631
Aspergillus versicolor	1	1	1	1	1
Aureobasidium pullulans	754	1273	5036	431	2288
Chaetomium globosum	49	2	21	14	51
Cladosporium sphaerospermum	2464	1758	2647	578	1119
Eurotium Group	512	409	762	173	224
Paecilomyces variotii	31	11	174	82	148
Penicillium brevicompactum	39	14	48	1	1
Penicillium corylophilum	1	1	1	1	36
Penicillium Group 2	1	1	1	1	1
Penicillium purpurogenum	1	1	1	1	3
Penicillium spinulosum	1	1	1	1	1
Penicillium variabile	12	4	37	16	95
Scopulariopsis brevicaulis	4	18	2	1	10
Scopulariopsis chartarum	1	1	1	1	1
Stachybotrys chartarum	1	1	11	1	1
Trichoderma viride	10	5	16	135	64
Wallemia sebi	75	43	250	42	57
Sum of the logs group 1	**32.66**	**29.32**	**39.05**	**27.88**	**33.39**
Group 2					
Acremonium strictum	1	1	4	1	1
Alternaria alternata	1	22	841	72	159
Aspergillus ustus	252	62	88	138	392
Cladosporium cladosporioides-1	611	502	1820	556	453
Cladosporium cladosporioides-2	19	3	12	6	17
Cladosporium herbarum	36	12	619	42	86
Epicoccum nigrum	20	16	499	19	95
Mucor Group	25	6	8	3	7
Penicillium chrysogenum Type 2	112	114	37	43	400
Rhizopus stolonifer	7	21	45	1	21
Sum of the logs group 2	**13.62**	**14.24**	**19.93**	**14.05**	**18.1**
ERMI values	**19.0**	**15.1**	**19.1**	**13.8**	**15.3**

Table C4. Bulk paint/matrix lead results for AFSHS

Sample location	Pb (µg/g)*	LOD (µg/g)	LOQ (µg/g)
April 19, 2005			
Room 403 under window sill	68.1	0.51	1.71
4th floor hallway outside wall	904.0	0.18	0.603
4th floor stairwell (even side)	11.4	0.37	1.24
Room 325 wall under window	1670	1.2	4.11
Room 325 window sill	1410	1.3	4.20
Room 321 wall by teacher's desk	1660	0.56	1.86
May 24, 2005			
Room 205 loose ceiling paint	1730	1.0	3.47

*Micrograms per gram total weight

Table C5. Culturable fungi in air sampling results for AFSHS

Sample location	Air volume per replicate (liters)	Average colony count (CFU/m³)*	Fungal identification, by rank
Room 420	141.5	246	Cladosporium Penicillium Basidiomycetes yeasts sterile fungi Alternaria alternata Botrytis cinerea Aspergillus glaucus Tritirachium
Room 316	141.5	321	Cladosporium Penicillium Aspergillus niger Aspergillus versicolor Aspergillus ochraceus Syncephalastrum sterile fungi yeasts Rhizopus stolonifer
Room 427	141.5	1000	Cladosporium Penicillium Alternaria alternata Epicoccum nigrum sterile fungi yeasts Basidiomycetes Aspergillus fumigatus Aspergillus sp. Fusarium
Room 205	141.5	888	Cladosporium Penicillium Aspergillus sp. Basidiomycetes sterile fungi yeasts Curvularia Epicoccum nigrum
Outside main entrance	141.5	1179	Cladosporium Penicillium Alternaria alternata sterile fungi yeasts Epicoccum nigrum Aureobasidium pullulans Fusarium

*Colony forming units per cubic meter (average of three replicates)

Table C6. Fungal spores in air using spore traps for AFSHS

Sampling location	Sample volume (liters)	Average total fungal structure (count/m³)*	Fungal identification by rank
Room 420	75	98	*Cladosporium>Basidiospores>Aspergillus/Pencillium-*like*>Ascospores*>Hyphal Fragments*> Ganoderma*
Room 316	75	338	*Aspergillus/Pencillium* like*>Cladosporium> Basidiospores>Ascospores>Mxyomycetes*>Hyphal Fragments*>Ulocladium*
Room 427	75	1911	*Cladosporium>Aspergillus/Pencillium-*like*> Basidiospores>Ascospores*>Hyphal Fragments*> Ganoderma>Epicoccum>Myxomycetes>Alternaria>Torula>Curvularia>Cercospora>Piuthomyces> Bipolaris/Dreschlera*
Room 205	75	1311	*Cladosporium>Basidiospores>Aspergillus/Pencillium-*like*>Ascospores*>Hyphal Fragments*> Myxomycetes> Alternaria>Ganoderma> Bipolaris/Dreschlera*
Outside main entrance	75	4000	*Cladosporium>Ascospores>Basidiospores> Alternaria>Aspergillus/Pencillium* like*>*Hyphal Fragments*>Epicocuum>Myxomycetes>Ganoderma>Cercospora>Periconia>Pithomyces>Polythrincium>Curvularia>Pestalotiopsis>Bipolaris/Dreschlera> Chaetomium>Curvularia*

*Count per cubic meter of air

Table C7. Microscopic sticky tape sample results for WHHS

Sample location	Genera	Amount of growth*
Room 102 – back wall in closet – evidence of chronic leakage	None	N/A†
Room 102 – back wall in closet – evidence of chronic leakage	Hyphae – unidentified genera	Trace
Room 102 – back wall in closet – evidence of chronic leakage	*Aspergillus/Penicillium*-like spores Hyphae – unidentified genera	A Few Trace
Room 103 – side wall in classroom – evidence of chronic leakage	None	N/A
Room -103 – rug sample – chronic leak pattern	None	N/A
Library – window leak	None	N/A
Library – shelving that had mold remediation completed	None	N/A
Room 333 – evidence of roof leak	None	N/A

*Massive>numerous>many>a few>trace
†Not applicable

Table C8. Fungal spore equivalents in air identified by MSQPCR for WHHS

Sample locations	Room 102	Room 103	Library	Room 271	Outside
Sampling time	8:28 a.m. – 2:09 p.m.	8:42 a.m. – 2:11 p.m.	8:58 a.m. – 2:14 p.m.	9:32 a.m. – 2:23 p.m.	9:40 a.m. – 2:26 p.m.
Fungal ID (SE/m^3)*					
Aspergillus fumigatus	ND†	ND	34	ND	35
Aspergillus niger	ND	ND	7	ND	ND
Cladosporium cladosporioides-1	1	4	ND	ND	ND
Eurotium (Asp.) amstelodami‡	ND	61	20	ND	210
Penicillium brevicompactum	ND	ND	ND	23	13
Penicillium chrysogenum	ND	ND	5	ND	ND

*Spore equivalent per cubic meter of air
†None detected
‡Detected in field blank

Table C9. Culturable air sample results for WHHS

Sample location	Air volume per replicate (liters)	Average colony count (CFU/m³)*	Fungal identification, by rank
Room 333	85	92	*Cladosporium* *Penicillium* *Epicoccum nigrum* *Aureobasidium pullalans*
Room 334	85	103	*Basidiomycetes* *Cladosporium* *Penicillium* *Yeasts* *Aspergillus niger* *Aspergillus sydowii* *Aspergillus versicolor* *Chrysosoporium pannorum* *Epicoccum nigrum*
Library	85	159	*Basidiomycetes* *Penicillium* sterile fungi yeasts *Aspergillus versicolor* *Fusarium* sp. *Phoma* sp. *Rhodotorula mucilaginosa*
Room 102	85	8	*Cladosporium* *Aspergillus caesitosus*
Room 260	85	12	Sterile fungi Yeasts
Outside main entrance	85	140	*Basidiomycetes* *Cladosporium* *Penicillium* yeasts sterile fungi Alternaria alternata *Aspergillus fumigatus* *Aspergillus nidulans* *Aspergillus versicolor* *Epicoccum nigrum*

*Colony forming units per cubic meter (average of three replicates). Sample results corrected for multiple impacts.

Table C10. Fungal spores in air using spore traps for WHHS

Sampling location	Sample volume (liters)	Total fungal structure (count/m³)*	Fungal identification by rank
Room 333	75	187	*Cladosporium> Aspergillus/Pencillium*-like> Hyphal Fragments> *Basidiospores> Pithomyces> Mxyomycetes>Rusts*
Room 334	75	373	*Aspergillus/Pencillium*-like> *Basidiospores> Epicocuum> Ganoderma>Mxyomycetes>*Hyphal Fragments
Library	75	253	*Aspergillus/Pencillium*-like> *Basidiospores>*Hyphal Fragments> *Myxomycetes>Cladosporium> Curvularia*
Room 102	75	27	*Basidiospores>* Hyphal Fragments
Room 260	75	93	*Aspergillus/Pencillium*-like> *Basidiospores> Pithomyces*
Outside Main Entrance	75	520	*Basidiospores> Aspergillus/Pencillium*-like> *Ascospores> Cladosporium>*Hyphal Fragments>Pollen

*Count per cubic meter of air

ACKNOWLEDGMENTS AND AVAILABILITY OF REPORT

The Hazard Evaluations and Technical Assistance Branch (HETAB) of the National Institute for Occupational Safety and Health (NIOSH) conducts field investigations of possible health hazards in the workplace. These investigations are conducted under the authority of Section 20(a)(6) of the Occupational Safety and Health Act of 1970, 29 U.S.C. 669(a)(6) which authorizes the Secretary of Health and Human Services, following a written request from any employer or authorized representative of employees, to determine whether any substance normally found in the place of employment has potentially toxic effects in such concentrations as used or found. HETAB also provides, upon request, technical and consultative assistance to federal, state, and local agencies; labor; industry; and other groups or individuals to control occupational health hazards and to prevent related trauma and disease.

The findings and conclusions in this report are those of the authors and do not necessarily represent the views of NIOSH. Mention of any company or product does not constitute endorsement by NIOSH. In addition, citations to websites external to NIOSH do not constitute NIOSH endorsement of the sponsoring organizations or their programs or products. Furthermore, NIOSH is not responsible for the content of these websites. All Web addresses referenced in this document were accessible as of the publication date.

This report was prepared by Gregory Thomas, Nancy Clark Burton, Charles Mueller, and Elena Page of HETAB, Division of Surveillance, Hazard Evaluations and Field Studies. Industrial hygiene field assistance was provided by Srinivas Durgam, Andrea Markey, Rob McCleery, and Perianan Periakaruppan. Medical field assistance was provided by Judith Eisenberg and Marilyn Radke. Analytical support was provided by Ronnee N. Andrews, Chemical Exposure Monitoring Branch, Division of Applied Research and Technology, and EMLab P&K Laboratories, Cherry Hill, New Jersey. Assistance with the ERMI analysis was provided by Steven Vesper, U.S. Environmental Protection Agency. Health communication assistance was provided by Stefanie Evans. Editorial assistance was provided by Ellen Galloway. Desktop publishing was performed by Robin Smith.

Copies of this report have been sent to employee and management representatives at the New Orleans Public School District, Walnut Hills High School, the state health department, and the Occupational Safety and Health Administration Regional Office. This report is not copyrighted and may be freely reproduced. The report may be viewed and printed at http://www.cdc.gov/niosh/hhe/. Copies may be purchased from the National Technical Information Service at 5825 Port Royal Road, Springfield, Virginia 22161.